EAT *the* BERRIES

EAT *the* BERRIES

Weight Loss *for* Busy Moms

Jaime Hernandez, M.A.

NEW YORK

LONDON • NASHVILLE • MELBOURNE • VANCOUVER

Eat the Berries

Weight Loss for Busy Moms

© 2020 Jamie Hernandez, M.A.

Published in New York, New York, by Morgan James Publishing in partnership with Difference Press. Morgan James is a trademark of Morgan James, LLC. www.MorganJamesPublishing.com

ISBN 9781642793307 paperback
ISBN 9781642793314 eBook
Library of Congress Control Number: 2018912809

Cover Design by:
Rachel Lopez
www.r2cdesign.com

Interior Design by:
Christopher Kirk
www.GFSstudio.com

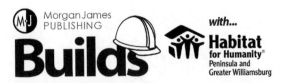

Morgan James is a proud partner of Habitat for Humanity Peninsula and Greater Williamsburg. Partners in building since 2006.

Get involved today! Visit
MorganJamesPublishing.com/giving-back

Dedication

I dedicate this book to all the moms out there who work so hard every day to raise our future and to Ashtyn, Marcus, Maxon, and Autumn for allowing me to do the best job in the world. And to D, for loving me and never giving up.

Table of Contents

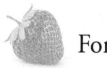

Foreword

In my opinion, the best-written books share timeless messages but are crafted in an original way. Jamie integrates her holistic outlook on life and healing in this sincere and well-thought-out approach to weight loss for moms. What immediately captivated me about this book is Jamie's authenticity. She is speaking from her heart, she is *telling you like it is*—and I hope you are listening. Talented coach, inspired writer, and wise young woman, Jamie has overcome many obstacles in her own life, and I know you will learn much from her.

Especially on point is the revelation that as a mom, you must come first! For many years, I had an extremely robust counseling and hypnotherapy practice in Southern California. Many parents booked consultations to discuss getting their kids (mainly teenagers) into therapy. Inevitably, after about fifteen minutes, it became clear that they were going to have to take their place in the chair before the kids. Parents impact their children from their own behavior, whether it is apparent or not. Children learn from your actions, so when you make *them* more important than your well-being, that is not a healthy message.

I came full circle to my own path of self-care and nourishment from having practically ruined my health in a period of intense stress and challenge. Having been considered a world-class expert in the subconscious mind and hypnotherapy, and deeply committed to a spiritual path, I finally realized that I had neglected the body. This brings to mind a meme I saw a few years ago on Facebook, the text of which was "If you don't take care of your body, where else will you live?"

The mind-body-spirit approach is the foundation of everything we teach at the Natural Wellness Academy. It is beyond gratifying to see how Jamie is carrying this message to the most important people the world—moms! *You* are the role models for a new generation. You are the givers of life, love, and encouragement. The analogy of "pouring from the full cup" is priceless.

In holism, the idea is that everything is connected and cannot operate at optimal levels without the interdependence of all the parts. The excellence of this book is how Jamie weaves in self-image and self-talk, as well as the need to develop a deeper connection to your spiritual self. All of these are interconnected to the issue of your weight. As you balance these different areas of your life, your body can naturally find a healthy medium and you will be inspired to make healthier, positive, life-affirming choices.

Whether you want to break a persistent negative habit, such as overeating, or create a life-affirming one, such as a regular exercise program, the secret lies in making the new behavior *second nature* to you. I hope that you embrace the wisdom in this book and create the most wonderful habit you can mirror to your loved ones—self-love.

As Jamie has discovered through her own journey and through working with her coaching clients, we need to learn to like ourselves enough to give our bodies the proper care they need. Losing weight or getting into shape should not be motivated by what others may think or how they may view us— it's about honoring ourselves and recognizing the spark of the divine within each of us. Imagine the power of mirroring such an enlightened perspective to your cherished children!

Wishing you a wonderful journey,

LindaJoy Rose, PhD

www.NaturalWellnessAcademy.org

Chapter One

You Are Here, You Can Do This!

"The greatest wealth is health."
– Virgil

So, let me guess. You got married (yay!) or got pregnant (woo-hoo!), and then after the honeymoon phase or the newly-wed phase or the babymoon phase or the "I have a newborn and I feel #blessed and complete" phase, you are here wondering, "What about ME?" And it's a very valid question to ask.

I'm guessing you chose this book because you don't feel or look the way you used to or want to, or because you want to lose weight that you put on from pregnancy or lack of self-care after becoming a mom, or both. Maybe you feel lost in your own body and your own life. You are not alone!

Mothering is a full-time, 24/7/365 job. For real. How do you get from devoting yourself to your child to finding the balance necessary to care for yourself as well? This is the question I get asked by so many moms who are in the same boat as you.

I have moms in my weight loss program who meet me for personal training or coaching and say it's the first time they have ever left their child. I see moms who say they used to work out every day before having kids and now they can't remember the last time they exercised their bodies. I see moms who make sure all of their kids' nutritional needs are met, but they eat tortilla chips and drink soda all day. Moms are the most powerful, resourceful, determined people on this planet. All you need to do is tap into those qualities that make you an amazing, devoted mom and turn them inward.

So here you are, wanting to make yourself a priority and lose weight. And here are some of the possible reasons you haven't done it. You may believe that you don't have time. *You Do*. You may believe that you don't have the energy. *You Do*. You may believe that you can wait until your kids are much older to take care of yourself. *You Can't*. You may believe you can't lose the weight; you have tried, you are tired, and nothing works. *Not True*.

You do have time. You do have the energy. You cannot afford to put your health on hold. You can lose the weight. You are a mom. You made a child. You birthed that child. You fed that child. You got up at night with that child. You are raising that child to be an amazing human being. *You* are amazing. *You* can do anything. Even this. Especially this.

Chapter Two

My Journey to Self-Care

"You cannot pour from an empty cup."
– Unknown

I have four kids. Yes, four (most people's responses include wide eyes, an "O" shaped mouth, and the word "Four!?"). Yes, four. Apparently that's considered a lot in this day and age. My oldest was born in 2008. I was twenty-nine years old. She was my world. I spent every day making sure that all of her needs were met. I made homemade baby food. I took her to baby gym classes, swimming lessons, playdates, and so on. She had it made! When she was two years old, I had my second. Then, things got a little more daunting. I started to feel overwhelmed, and I was only halfway done! Over the next four years, I would have two more. Somewhere in there, I lost myself. Somewhere in there, I stopped paying attention to myself and my needs. Somehow, mommy guilt surfaced and took over.

At this point, my best friend told me a story that changed me. It went something like *You know, every time I go to the grocery store, I spend five dollars on a carton of organic strawberries for my kids. Then I lovingly rinse them, cut them up into small pieces, and put them on their plates. But you know what? I never eat the strawberries. Not one. I give them all to my kids. I want a strawberry!* So why didn't she eat a strawberry? Because she thought it was more important for her kids to have them. It's more important for her kids to be healthy and eat the expensive five-dollar strawberries. When did this happen? When did we become our last priority?

When my kids were babies and toddlers, I felt guilty if I did anything that did not involve being with them or that wouldn't contribute to their well-being. Therefore, no exercise, because that would take away from time I could be paying attention to my kids. No preparing healthy snacks and meals for myself—I only had time to make those for my kids. No relaxing or reading a book when they were awake—nope, I had to be right there beside them, teaching them something. My health suffered. I felt tired and drained all of the time. I felt stressed and my patience was at an all-time low. I spent all my time trying to be a "good mom," but I felt like a "horrible mom."

Everyone said, "Enjoy this time while it lasts, they grow up so fast!" This went through my head. Every. Single. Day. How could I waste any of this precious time with them? I didn't know what to do. My thought process went something like, "I had these kids, I'm responsible for them, they won't be little forever, and when they are older, I can focus on myself." So I focused on them. I ignored myself.

Then, somewhere between children numbers three and four, I realized that I had a passion for (was obsessed with) natural health and nutrition. I was lucky enough to stumble across the Natural Wellness Academy, which is run by my dedicated mentor, Dr. LindaJoy Rose. I discovered that I could become a certified holistic health and life coach in nine to twelve months and could have a practice that would help others learn how to live a healthy lifestyle. I was a vegetarian and did OK when it came to diet, but like my friend, I was a little obsessive about making sure my kids ate nutritious, clean foods. After seeing them munching on broccoli, people always asked, "How do you get them to eat that?" I thought, "I can help parents get their kids to eat healthy foods. This is perfect!"

Twelve months later I finished my program, and I was inspired and excited. I was finally doing something for me. I started marketing myself as a parent coach to get kids to eat healthier. Moms were coming to me asking for help, but after working with several clients, I had an "aha" moment. Just like my friend, these mom clients were also not eating the berries.

Moms were eating fast food, junk food, anything on-the-go food, because that's how they prioritized their health. Their kids saw this and wanted to imitate it. So, that's when I realized, healthy moms = healthy kids. I have to start with moms. This is when the law of attraction took hold of my life. As soon as I had this realization, I started getting tons of new clients, moms who wanted to lose weight and take care of themselves and their families. This was my calling! I can help kids by helping their moms. I can help dads and entire families by helping moms. Moms are in charge. Moms set the example. Moms run families. Healthy moms = healthy families!

For me, this career aspiration was what pushed me into the realm of self-care. Once I decided to take this time for myself to pursue a career, I realized that prioritizing myself made me a better parent. I started to make myself healthy food, and I began exercising. Yep, I dropped my kids off at the childcare at the gym, felt a slight pang of guilt if they cried when I walked away, but still went to the workout room and did it. And when I picked them up they were happy, and so was I. I was eating the berries!

For most of my clients, it's being tired of carrying around the extra weight and feeling bad about it. It's not knowing how to start, what to do, and how to not feel guilty doing it once you figure it out. But once you start, you are unstoppable! You will notice positive changes in all areas of your life! You will lose weight, feel better, look healthier, be happier, and your kids and loved ones will all benefit from this new you!

Chapter Three

Get Excited!

*"If you want to live a life you've never lived, you have to
do things you have never done."*
– Jen Sincero, *You Are a Bada***

So at this point, you are probably wondering, "How is this book going to help me lose weight?" I'm now going to share that secret with you. After working with many clients just like you, I have discovered what makes some succeed right away, while others have to try harder over longer periods of time. Ready? The ones who achieve success that lasts are those who are in true alignment with their weight loss goals in body, mind, and spirit. They are *really, truly* ready on all levels of their being. They are ready to take care of their bodies, they are ready to change their thoughts, and they are ready to use everything that the universe is offering them to achieve this goal. Therefore, I have set up this book in a way that helps you succeed in this same way.

Your weight loss journey can be a miserable experience in which you feel deprived and irritated every single day. Or it can be one of the most powerful and transformative life experiences you have ever had. I want to guide you to the second choice. Just like every other challenge in life, your weight loss journey can be a journey to self-discovery. Why have you put on this weight, and what does it mean to lose it? Why are you worth it? What are you meant to learn from it? How is it going to make you a better person and mom? This book is your guide not only to weight loss but also to reaching a place of self-love and being the strong, confident woman you are!

First, I will teach you how to care for your body through diet, exercise, and implementing a realistic plan that is achievable and maintainable. Second, I will help you determine whether or not your thoughts are aligned with this plan, and if they aren't, I will teach you how to change them so that they are. Finally, I will make you understand that the universe is on your side. You can tap into whatever spirituality means to you to help you succeed. This is the holistic approach. This is the key to success.

You are amazing, *you* are important, *you* deserve to be healthy and happy and joyful. *You*, the mom, are the core of the family, the example for your kids, the caretaker, the nurturer, the one they look up to. *You* are so many amazing things. As Jen Sincero says, *You* are a bada** (awesome book). So, what about you?

How will you love yourself and take care of your amazing self? I truly believe that the greatest wealth is health (Virgil), and this book can bring you both. You will be overflowing with the wealth that is health. You can lose that weight. You can continue to be an amazing mom. Get excited!

Chapter Four

~~Diet~~ Nourishment

"The food you eat can either be the safest and most
powerful form of medicine, or the slowest form of poison."
– Ann Wigmore

ood. We love it. We hate that we love it. This, my mom friends, has to change. Food is necessary. Food is life! Food gives us the nutrition we need to not just survive but thrive. It's time to start eating the foods that will make you thrive—have more energy, lose weight, feel confident, feel calm. The old adage "You are what you eat" is in fact true. If you eat junk, you will feel horrible. If you eat clean, nutritious foods, you will feel alive.

So what's the deal with this chapter being called "nourishment" instead of "diet" or "food"? The deal is, you *must* have a positive relationship with food in order for weight loss to become your reality. The word *diet* automatically conjures the idea of restriction and deprivation. You have to imagine yourself eating nutritious foods and really enjoying it. Food is not the enemy. Food is amazing. Food is life. The right food nourishes your body, mind, and soul. Nourishment = a nutrient-dense diet. When your diet primarily consists of nutrient-dense foods, weight loss naturally occurs. Nourish your body with nutrients. That's it.

Calories

Honestly, I'm not really a proponent of calorie counting, and here is why. You can eat very few calories in a day, but eat foods that are not nourishing your body. I prefer to focus on nutrient-dense foods that are naturally low in calories that you can eat in abundance. So what are these nutrients I'm talking about? I'm glad you asked!

Macronutrients

Macronutrients are what most people focus on when looking at the composition of their food, and refer to protein, fat, and carbohydrates. There are various diets that recommend different ratios and amounts of these macronutrients for weight loss.

All of these macronutrients are essential. Some would say carbohydrates are not; however, carbohydrates are in most foods, including fruits and vegetables, so you cannot eliminate them completely. Nutrient-dense carbohydrates contain an abundance of fiber, which is beneficial for weight loss. Whole-food carbohydrates are heart-healthy and a fantastic source of energy. Sure, eating too many carbs, especially highly processed ones, can cause weight gain. However, anything in excess can be detrimental. Eating a moderate amount of whole-food carbohydrates, such as rice, oatmeal, and quinoa, will nourish your body with essential nutrients, give you energy, and assist with weight loss.

Speaking of excess, our society is extremely fixated on protein. Protein is absolutely necessary for health and survival. However, it's again a nutrient that should be consumed in moderate, appropriate amounts. Your body can process only so much protein at a time, and the rest is turned into fat. Excess protein is stored as fat, ladies! Therefore, high-protein diets can not only cause weight gain (or lack of weight loss), but over the long term can cause strain on the kidneys or heart (especially when consuming animal protein).

According to www.nutrition.com, "to get your personal protein 'RDA' (recommended daily amount), multiply the number 0.36 by your weight in pounds. (For a sedentary 150-pound woman, that would be 54 grams.) Double it if you're very active."

Fat

Fat got a bad rap many years ago, but now we realize that good fats are beneficial for health. Unhealthy fats—such as those found in dairy products and other animal products, fried foods, and processed snack foods—can lead to heart disease, cancer, and other chronic diseases, as well as weight gain. Healthy fats—such as those found in fish, nuts and seeds, and avocados—are fats you should include in your diet in moderation. Eating healthy fats will make you feel full, and therefore you will consume fewer calories while improving your heart health and metabolism. They also help your body absorb and process important nutrients, and they even boost serotonin levels in your brain, making you feel happy! Fat is also needed to burn calories, as it provides twice the amount of energy as carbohydrates and protein. Don't fear good fats!

Overall, your best bet is to focus on a balanced, whole-food nourishment plan that does not overly emphasize, or cut out, entire macronutrient groups.

Micronutrients

Micronutrients are generally not what people consider when planning their diet, but they should! Micronutrients include all of the vitamin and minerals in our food. Even food labels only list a few of them on the box! Micronutrients include minerals such as iron, sodium, iodine, and zinc, to name a few. Vitamins—A, C, K, D, and all of the B varieties, among many others—are also micronutrients.

There are tools out there, such as Dr. Mercola's Cronometer (available to use for free on his website or you can download the app for a few dollars), that track the calorie and fat content of the food you eat, as well as all macro and micronutrients. For me and my clients, this is a much better food-tracking method. It encourages you to eat nutrient-dense foods and is motivating, as you watch your nutrition intake rise all day long when you enter your food!

Water

How much easier does it get than drinking water? The truth is, most Americans are dehydrated. They think they shouldn't drink unless they are thirsty. However, thirst can come in the form of feeling hungry, which leads to eating when you are in fact thirsty, not hungry. In fact, a University of Washington study showed that participants who were dieting stopped hunger pangs almost 100 percent of the time by drinking a glass of water. What?! It's easy, it's free, it's everywhere. It's a simple habit to add. Not only is it an appetite suppressant, but it gives you energy and healthy skin, aids with digestion, and cleanses your kidneys. There is absolutely no reason to not drink more water, so this is something you need to add to your weight loss plan.

Eat Whole, Be Whole

What are whole foods? Whole foods are any foods in their natural form, just as they come from the earth. Some examples are fruits, vegetables, eggs, nuts, seeds, beans, and whole grains, such as rice, quinoa, and barley. Unprocessed meat, such as chicken breasts and steak or other beef cuts, are generally considered whole foods. Meats such as ground beef or chicken are more processed, and obviously things like chicken fingers and hot dogs are not considered whole foods, as they come from a box.

Aiming for a diet that is 90 percent whole foods is ideal. That means 90 percent of your food does not come from a box. If you eat 90 percent whole foods, you will lose weight and feel amazing. I usually start my clients at a 60/40 or 70/30 whole-to-processed foods ratio and build up to 90/10 during our work together.

This plan does not mean that you never get to eat pizza or cupcakes or whatever your favorite treat foods are. Attempting to eliminate those foods forever will be like trying to not pay attention to the big pink cupcake in the room—it's all you will think about! Instead it means eating those things sparingly. Cheat meals are a useful part of any nourishment plan because if you try to deprive yourself of the things you love, you will rebel. It's okay to eat a cupcake once or twice a month. It's not serving your health goals to eat one every day. It's about having a diet that is mostly nutrient-dense foods, which is where the 90/10 comes in. The 10 percent allows you to have those comfort foods you don't want to live without. But chances are, when your taste buds are retrained to enjoy the taste of real, whole foods, those other things just won't be as appealing. The other good news is, whole foods are more filling per calorie than processed foods, so you can eat less to feel full!

Here are examples of whole foods you should include in your diet:

- Water
- Fruits and vegetables
- Beans
- Nuts and seeds
- Eggs
- Herbs and Spices
- Olive oil (not heated)
- Coconut oil

Olive oil does not have a high smoke point, and therefore becomes toxic when heated and used for cooking. However, it's great for dressings and dips. Coconut oil has a higher smoke point, and so does avocado oil, so these are ideal for cooking.

Bio-Individuality

Bio-individuality is the idea that there is not a one-size-fits-all diet for any person. Each body is different, and responds differently to different foods and ways of eating. You have probably heard someone say how awesome the Paleo diet is for weight loss, or the plant-based diet, or the macro diet. That doesn't mean it will be awesome for you.

The journey of discovering how your body responds to certain foods is crucial for weight loss. Some people need more protein, some need less. Some benefit from eating more carbs, some people gain weight when they eat more carbs. The point is, don't feel frustrated if you try the amazing diet your neighbor or BFF told you about and you don't have the same results. Pay attention to your body and how it responds to what you eat. It's an art that can be developed with time and patience. But it's so worth it!

Many times, my clients start with an elimination diet or a gut-healing diet (see the next section). Eliminating highly reactive foods and slowly adding them back in is invaluable, not only for weight loss, but also for disease prevention and lifelong health. Inflammation is pervasive in our bodies today and is being discovered to be the source of diseases such as heart disease, cancer, and diabetes, as well as GI and autoimmune diseases. Eliminating inflammatory foods (which are mostly processed foods) will lead not only to weight loss but also to more energy to spend with your family!

Gut Health and Healing

I start my weight loss program with a gut-healing protocol. I find that weight loss happens much more quickly and easily after clients heal their gut. A typical protocol is three to four weeks, in which time I typically see weight loss of ten to twenty pounds. Here is why it's important. Our gut is made up of 100 trillion microorganisms. I don't even know how to comprehend that! The human gut contains ten times more bacteria than all the human cells in the entire body. We are more bacteria than cells! The fact that our body is so heavily comprised of bacteria shows how much of an impact it can have on our overall health and wellness.

Gut health, or lack thereof, has been linked to everything from cancer and heart disease to anxiety and depression. An unhealthy gut leads to inflammation in the body, which leads to chronic disease and autoimmune diseases. Healing your gut is so important for not only weight loss but also lifelong physical and mental health. Poor gut health is a result of eating foods low in nutritional value, such as processed foods and sugars, as well as environmental toxins and medications.

Gut-healing protocols involve removing all toxins and highly reactive foods, such as gluten, dairy, corn, sugar, soy, and all processed food. After this, you add in highly digestible foods such as rice, beans, lean proteins, and vegetables, as well as supplements such as probiotics and digestive enzymes and fermented foods and drinks. Finally, the highly reactive foods are slowly added back in so that you can notice any reactions your body has. When you are aware of your food sensitivities, you can decide if you want to continue to consume those foods.

Several fantastic things occur with clients during the gut-healing protocol. Weight loss is the obvious one, but clients also report having more energy, feeling more emotionally and mentally clear, and no longer having cravings for sugar and processed foods. Most clients don't want the protocol to end because they feel so good! After completing the protocol, they realize that they can get through cravings, and they learn to enjoy the taste of real, whole foods. Through this process, you can retrain your taste buds to love the foods that are good for you. This, combined with the motivation you get from losing weight, is why I recommend healing your gut at the beginning of any weight loss plan.

I worked with Penelope (client names have been changed for privacy) for many months, and although she had improved her diet and implemented an exercise plan, she was stuck when it came to weight. She was feeling better and was more energetic, but the lack of weight loss was discouraging her; she wanted to fall back to old habits. At this point, she agreed to do a gut-healing cleanse with me. Within two months of starting and completing the gut-healing protocol, she was down twenty pounds—her goal! That's when I changed my program to begin with gut healing. The term "heal your gut, heal your life" is in fact true! I have included two of my favorite gut healing books in the recommended reading section.

Green Smoothies

This was not meant to be a recipe book; however, I am known in my community as "the smoothie girl" because not only do I love smoothies but also talking to people about smoothies and teaching them how to experience their benefits. This love started when my oldest daughter was a toddler and I could not get her to eat any vegetables. My awesome, super-healthy, hippy vegan brother told me about green smoothies, and low and behold, she loved them! I would make her smoothies every day with various fruits and vegetables like kale, spinach, cucumbers, carrots, and beets. Then I discovered that I loved them too! When I drank them, my digestion was better, I had more energy, and I was less hungry. I also experienced fewer sugar cravings. When you drink one first thing in the morning, you are starting your day with something that is so good for you that you will want to continue making healthy choices as the day goes on.

Green smoothies are any smoothies that contain leafy greens, such as spinach, kale, romaine lettuce, collard greens, chard, or even parsley. Greens are one of the most nutrient-dense foods on the planet, and most people don't eat enough of them. And even if they did, you would have to chew a bite of salad 100 times to break it down enough to get all of the nutrients you get from liquifying them in a smoothie!

This is also where I start with my clients, and green smoothies are actually included in every single day of the gut-healing protocol! Adding one green smoothie a day will truly make a big difference in your health. If you have never had one, I know you might be hesitant, but you have to trust me. I have been making these nutrition powerhouse drinks for nine years, so I have it down; these recipes are good!

So if you have been wondering where to start with improving your diet, this is it: green smoothies and gut healing. You can find lots of recipes online and on Pinterest, but here are a few of my favorites:

Jamie's Go-To

　　1 cup spinach
　　¼ large cucumber, diced

1 cup frozen pineapple

water or coconut water

Minty Mojito

½ cup spinach

¼ large cucumber, diced

¼ cup parsley or 1 TB fresh mint leaves

1 cup frozen pineapple

juice of ½ lime

water or coconut water

Banana Split

½ cup spinach

1 banana

½ cup frozen strawberries

½ cup frozen pineapple

Water or coconut water

Mindful Eating

Mindfulness is a hot, hot topic right now, and for good reason! In fact, I dedicated a whole chapter of this book to mindfulness. For the purposes of this chapter, mindful eating is worth practicing.

As a mom, I'm sure you have had the experience of eating on-the-go or even at the dinner table, as fast as you possibly can. I'm guilty of both! However, part of developing this positive relationship with food *and* discovering what foods work best for your body is practicing mindful eating. Well, what the bleep does that mean?

Mindful eating means slowing down, chewing slowly, allowing your food to nourish you, and noticing when you are full. When you are shoveling in your food, your brain doesn't have time to process the hunger signals. You will keep eating, even though you are actually full. Chewing thoroughly allows your body to break down the food with digestive enzymes that assist with digestion, allowing your body to absorb more of the nutrition it's receiving.

A good practice is to put your utensil down between each bite and don't pick it up again until you have swallowed your food. Chew your food, pay attention to how your stomach feels. Notice when you are full and stop eating. Give yourself permission to truly enjoy the food you are eating. Give your kids permission to eat slowly as well. It's not a race; it's an experience to be savored! Even if your baby or toddler is throwing his food on the floor, even if your five-year-old is complaining that she doesn't like it, be an example of calmly and mindfully enjoying this time. Mindful eating is a key component of weight loss. And sometimes, the simplest solution is the one that works! Eat slowly, put down your fork, chew, enjoy.

Why Moms Struggle with Healthy Eating

Being a mom is not for wimps. It's hard work. It's a lot of work. It's draining and time-consuming. It's easy to forget about you. But how can you expect your kids to eat healthy foods if they don't have a role model who shows them how to do so? We read parenting books and blogs and websites on how to be a "good mom." Being a good role model is being a good mom. If you want your kids to eat a healthy diet, you have to eat a healthy diet. Start with you.

I refer back to the berries. You are important. You are worth feeding a healthy diet to. You deserve a healthy body just as much as your kids do. Believe me when I tell you this!

It truly does not have to mean making gourmet meals that you see on Pinterest. It's just about buying clean, nutritious foods, even if they are on-the-go foods. It means weaning your taste buds off salty and sugary processed foods, and getting back to enjoying the taste of very basic, nutrient-dense foods. I work with my clients to simplify this process and take the pressure off.

Now What?

So, now you might be wondering, what do I do with this information? Knowledge is power. You now have the knowledge to start taking this step in the right direction when it comes to improving your diet. Heal your gut. Eat foods high in nutrients, which are whole foods. Minimize processed, boxed foods. Drink water. Practice mindful eating. Drink one green smoothie a day. It really is that simple! And if it doesn't seem as simple for you, you can definitely hire a coach, like me, to support you through the process.

Chapter Five

I Like to Move It, Move It

"Exercise is a celebration of what your body can do, not a punishment for what you ate."
— Unknown

Let's face it, if you want to lose weight, you have to exercise. You have to burn calories and build muscle to be your ideal weight. It's just part of the journey. However, I happen to think it's the best part!

Why don't you exercise? Most of my clients say, "I don't have time." It's about getting the kids ready for school then going to work in the morning or running errands or being with younger kids all day and then being exhausted at night. I get it. (Really, like I was there for a long time. I get it.) However, let me present an idea to you: exercise *is* fun! Exercise will make you feel alive in mind, body, and spirit. Exercise can happen, no matter what. In fact, one of my most vivid childhood memories is my mom putting an exercise record on the record player (I believe Jane

Fonda, but not sure) and doing her workout in our living room. And I did it with her, and I loved it. My mom did not spend every moment making sure I was learning something or entertained or taken care of in every way. She exercised, I saw it, and I learned that taking care of your body is important. My first few years as a parent were the only times in my life that I didn't work out regularly. And I have always felt that this memory was a big part of it. My mom was my hero, and if she exercised her body, then I thought I should, too.

That is why you are not being selfish or taking away from your children by committing to exercise. Good role model, remember?

Here are the other reasons:

Physical Benefits

If your goal is to lose weight, then you need to burn calories and build muscle. Walking twenty minutes on the treadmill once a day is not going to cut it, just being honest. If you aren't working out at all, then this is an acceptable place to start, but you will need to up your game after a week or two.

Strength training is also necessary for weight loss. Muscle burns fat all day long. When you build muscle, it is burning fat while you sleep! So, as a personal trainer giving general advice, I'm saying be sure your exercise routine includes strength training in some way, shape, or form, whether it's classes or machines at the gym or spending a little money on some weights and bands and finding videos that show you how to use them.

A good plan for weight loss is to work out at least four times a week. Each workout should contain strength training that focuses on one area of the body. So a sample weekly workout plan could be:

- Monday: 30 minutes on the treadmill, 20-minute strength-training for legs, 10 minutes of core/ab work
- Tuesday: 30 minutes speed walking or running outside, 20-minute strength training for arms, 10 minutes of core/ab work
- Wednesday: 30 minutes on elliptical, 10 minutes of core/ab work
- Thursday: Rest day
- Friday: 30 minutes on the treadmill, 20-minute strength-training for legs, 10 minutes of core/ab work
- Saturday: 30 minutes speed walking or running outside, 20-minute strength training for arms, 10 minutes of core/ab work
- Sunday: Rest day

You also need to stretch before and after each individual workout.

If this seems too time-consuming, you can find thirty-minute workouts that simultaneously focus on cardio, strength, and core, which is what I teach clients in my weight loss program. As a busy mom, I realize that getting the most bang for your time buck is important. Thirty minutes of intense exercise that focuses on all three is the most time-efficient way to burn calories, build strength, and lose weight!

People often feel frustrated when they start a strength-training program because they may not lose weight. But that's because muscle weighs more than fat, and you are often gaining muscle and losing fat, which is a good thing!

Strength training is especially important for women in preventing osteoporosis, as well as cancer, heart disease, and diabetes. *Really* think about this. These are very prevalent diseases in industrialized countries right now. What if you could do something fun, that made you a more present and energized mom, that would also give you health for years to come? Why would you choose to not do that?

Mental and Emotional Benefits

As moms, we can feel emotionally and mentally exhausted and drained much of the time. We give so much of our mental energy to our children and have little left for ourselves. This drain can certainly lead to feelings of depression or anxiety. The good news is exercise is a proven, natural way to overcome anxiety and depression! Even if you don't have a diagnosis of anxiety or depression, you will still reap the benefits. Regular exercise has been scientifically proven to make people feel calmer, more centered and focused, and happier. And I have seen it for myself. When I work with moms in my weight loss program, I see the smiles on their faces when they finish a workout. They text me later to tell me how energetic and positive they feel all day, all due to thirty minutes of exercise! Over the twelve weeks, I start to see joy and hope where I didn't before in these amazing moms. I see a sense of pride and accomplishment. During our online group workouts, sometimes their kids are running around in the background, and sometimes they wake up when their kids are still asleep. Sometimes they think they are too exhausted at the end of the day, but they do it anyway and never, ever regret it.

How Do I Work Out When I Have Kids?

So, there are the reasons why you should workout and here is the how. There are lots of different ways to make it happen.

The first step is figuring out when your ideal exercise time will be. Are you a person who is able to get up early—a morning person? Are you a person who has some time to kill in the afternoon, or do you have an energy spike in the evening before or after dinner? You have to fit it in somewhere, and you will if you make it a priority. Once you figure this out, here are four options for being a mom and creating an exercise routine:

1. Join a gym with childcare.

If you can afford to join your local YMCA or other gym with childcare, *just do it*. This was the best decision I ever made when my second child was a baby. I was able to take some time for myself and improve my health, while my kids got to socialize with other kids and play with different toys. Yes, they cried sometimes, and separation was sometimes hard. But guess what: years later, they have no memory of it, and they are completely fine. I remember when I would pick them up, I felt full of energy and a sense of calm and they could sense that! Taking that one hour to focus on me and my health was huge, not just for my physical well-being, but also for my mental and emotional health. This approach can also nurture your relationship with your significant other if you are able to do a workout together!

2. Hire a babysitter and go to the gym.

If your favorite class or gym does not offer childcare, find someone to come be with your kids and make it happen. When you return, you will feel refreshed and energized. I always thought of it like this: had I spent this last hour with my kids, I would likely be feeling drained, overwhelmed, and dare I say, bored, right now. Instead, I just took this hour to fuel my body with endorphins, and now I have the mindset and energy to be present and alive with my kids. Plus, they get to see that physical exercise is a priority!

An alternative to this is going when your significant other is home in the evening or on the weekends. Let he/she take over, and you get it done!

3. Work out at home.

This is why no one has an excuse. Regardless of your parental or financial status, as long as you have an internet connection, you can work out. At this point, because I am working full-time and have four kids with homework and activities, I work out at 5:30 a.m. in my home. I don't have time to go to the gym, even though I belong to a gym with childcare. I am a morning person, so I get up at 5:00 a.m. and oftentimes at least two of my kids are up with me. They know this is my workout time. I give them a little breakfast snack and a drink and, yes, the dreaded device, and I work out. Other times, they want to work out with me. They try to do the moves and they even cheer me on!

I pay for a subscription workout service, but even if you can't afford to do that, you can use YouTube or Amazon Prime or Netflix. You can also hire a virtual personal trainer—yes, this is a thing. If you have equipment at home, use it. Let your kids see you using it. Teach them about exercise and its benefits. Don't separate them from the process. They worship you. They learn from you. They will do what you do. Whatever your life circumstance is, you can work out. You will benefit. Your kids will benefit. It is a win-win.

4. Swap babysitting with a friend.

This is a great option that not only gives your kids a playdate but also holds you accountable! Ask a friend to babysit for you while you go to the gym, and offer the same to her. Don't let each other cancel or make excuses. This is really a win-win!

Make It Fun, Be Accountable

These are the two best tips for sustaining a workout regimen. You have so many fantastic options when it comes to working out! Whether you like to dance or do yoga or ballet or just straight up cardio and weights, you can find a class or video that fulfills your idea of fun. Try different things. Be adventurous! Go outside if you can and experience nature while you work out. Make it as fun and exciting as possible.

Accountability is extremely important for sticking to the consistent routine you need to achieve weight loss. The theory is that it takes twenty-one days to make and break habits. Therefore, you will need to work out consistently for three weeks to a month for it to become a habit. There are a few ways you can have accountability. One is to have a workout buddy. This is a great option because it's free and also because you have someone to work out with you. Find someone at your gym or even a friend who wants to come over to do videos with you at your house.

Another way is to hire a trainer. A personal trainer will not only push you to do your best, but you will also be more likely to show up for your workouts if you know someone is there expecting you. Many trainers often ask you to pay for missed sessions, which is another way to ensure attendance. Many of my clients say they did not feel like getting out of bed to work out, but they did it because they didn't want to let me down. Now, I know that by not working out, they are letting themselves down, not me, but whatever gets them there is fine with me. Like I mentioned before, even virtual training is a viable option now. I work with clients via the internet and can show them how to use their equipment while motivating them and ensuring they are being safe and have proper form.

One last option is hiring a health coach. I hold my coaching clients accountable by asking them to develop weekly workout plans and then sending them reminder/motivational texts and asking them to send me pictures of their workout. Accountability is very, very important for the first month of developing a new habit. It's worth the investment. Once it is a habit, the way you feel and the results you see will be your motivation.

Holistic Benefits

Here is what happens when you exercise. Exercise releases endorphins, which makes you feel happier and improves your mood and outlook. When you are happier, you are a more present and calm parent, and you are more likely to make other healthy choices. When you feel good on the inside, you will lose weight. You have to be in a place of self-love and joy to lose weight. Exercise will help to get you there. It lifts you up in mind, body, and spirit. It is worth it!

Chapter Six

Plan for Success

"Failing to plan is planning to fail."
– Alan Lakein

Whether or not you are a planner by nature, you need to plan to achieve weight loss. You just have to; trust me. Planning meals, snacks, and exercise is one of the very first habits I help new clients to establish. Because if you don't have a plan, you will fall back on old habits, which clearly did not work in your favor.

How to Plan Meals

A big part of losing weight and maintaining a healthy lifestyle is creating new habits. My role as a health coach is to help people through the process of establishing those new habits successfully. As I discussed in the last chapter, it typically takes about three weeks, or twenty-one days, to break and create habits, and I have found this to be true. My coaching packages are six weeks long, which allows me to have time to help clients create the habits and make sure they have the skills they need to maintain them.

Planning meals is one of the new habits you *need* to create. Like exercise, you may think you don't have time. However, once you do it consistently, you will find that it actually saves you time. By having a shopping list and meal plan, it takes away the guesswork of the week. Many clients create a two-, three-, or four-week rotation with meals that they repeat over and over. Once you have that down, it's less work for you!

The first step in meal planning is to decide what your shopping day will be. It is best to only shop once or twice per week, which will ultimately save you time. By planning, you don't have to go to the grocery store several times per week. You will have a list of what you need for the week, and you will do one big trip. Many stores offer delivery or pickup options, which can also save you time and money, since you won't give in to impulse purchases.

So, step one is determining what day each week that you will shop for groceries. Step two is to carve out a day and time that you will plan meals every week. Put it on your calendar. Make it just as important as a work meeting or Gymboree class or parent-teacher conference. This is one of the pillars of weight loss success. You must make it a priority.

Step three is doing it! There are lots of different ways to meal plan. Pinterest is a fantastic resource; in fact, I create Pinterest boards for all of my clients where I post healthy recipes to help them reach their goals. I generally try to choose recipes that contain similar ingredients for budget purposes. I also choose recipes that can be used as leftovers for lunch. You will also want to choose recipes that your kids like or that are easily adaptable as a meal for both you and your kids.

In general, focus on whole foods and make sure you are getting a good amount of vegetables. Here is a very general sample daily menu:

Breakfast

Green smoothie and

2 eggs or

Rice cakes or sprouted grain bread with raw nut butter or coconut oil or

Oatmeal or quinoa with nondairy milk and fruit

Mid-Morning Snack

Low-sugar protein bar or

Trail mix that contains nuts and dried fruit (a handful) or

Fruit and a handful of raw nuts or

Vegetables and hummus

Lunch

Dinner leftovers or
Salad that contains healthy fats and protein

Mid-Afternoon Snack

Smoothie—protein smoothie or green smoothie

Dinner

Lean protein (beans, tofu, fish, chicken) and vegetables or
whole grains (quinoa, brown rice, etc.) and vegetables

Evening snack

Warm lemon water to curb cravings

You can find plenty of recipes and ideas on Pinterest, and
I have several on my Pinterest profile at Whole Food & Spirit.

Planning workouts

I always ask clients to plan workouts just like they do
meals. Put them on your calendar and find someone to hold
you accountable. If you don't have a plan, you will keep putting
it off. It's easy to say "I don't have time today, but I'll definitely
do it tomorrow," if you don't have a solid plan. Whether you
are going to the gym or working out at home, plan your work-

outs at the same time you do your meal-planning each week. Decide what time you will put on that video or attend a class. Plan for success!

Sleep

Another part of planning and time management is planning for a good night's sleep. Sleep is very important for health and weight loss. When you are tired, you are more likely to choose the unhealthy comfort foods and you are definitely less likely to work out. Choose a time you will go to sleep every night and set an alarm on your phone for thirty minutes beforehand so you can start preparing. Set an alarm for the same time each weekday morning as well. All of my weight loss clients use my sleep hypnosis for deep, productive sleep that allows them to get up and work out and make healthy choices all day long! Claire was a weight loss client I worked with who didn't even realize how poor her sleep was until she started sleeping through the night, after which she finally had the energy to commit to a weight loss plan!

Planning is key for weight loss, just like it is for parenting. You plan swimming lessons, playdates, crafts, sporting events, etc., so you already know how to do it. Set the intention of planning for weight-loss success. It's more work at the beginning, but once you create habits, you no longer need to plan because those habits are established and become second nature. Take the time and effort in the beginning to set yourself up to succeed. It's so worth it!

Chapter Seven

You Are What You Think

"What you think, you become."
– Buddha

"Our body is really the product of our thoughts."
– Dr. John Hagelin

Are you ready? This is where the real work starts. How many times have you or someone you know tried to change their diet and exercise, but without lasting results? The next five chapters are your secret to weight-loss success: real, lasting weight loss and lifelong health and wellness. Because you are what you think. If you think that holding on to that weight is serving a purpose for you, you will not lose it. That thought is often held subconsciously, without your awareness. It's often something that stems from childhood or a traumatic experience. Whatever it is, you have to change your mind about it.

There are many ways you can tap into your subconscious to alter those self-sabotaging thoughts. Even if you don't have them or don't think you have them, you will still benefit from ensuring that your subconscious is on your side. One of my all-time favorite books is *You Are a Bada*** by Jen Sincero, and she devotes her entire first chapter to this, which is titled "My Subconscious Made Me Do It." There are so many powerful excerpts from this book, but here is one of my favorites on this particular topic:

> *"No matter what you say you want, if you've got an underlying subconscious belief that it's going to cause you pain or isn't available to you, you either A) Won't let yourself have it, or B) You will let yourself have it, but you'll be all f***ed up about it. And then you'll go off and lose it anyway."*

My weight-loss program includes hypnosis because I have always found more success with clients who use it. You are what you think, and you need to change your mind to change your life. Willpower isn't enough. Willpower comes from your conscious mind. Think of your mind as an iceberg. Your conscious mind, which is comprised of your thoughts and feelings that you are aware of, is represented by the tip of the iceberg. You can see it, but it's actually a very small part of the iceberg. Under the water, and not within your awareness, is the larger subconscious mind, which actually drives your behavior. Your subconscious mind is made up of all the thoughts and beliefs that you have collected over the years based on your experiences. They are the thoughts and beliefs that you are not aware of but that are driving your behaviors, for better or worse. According to Michael Bernard Beckwith, as quoted in *The Secret,* "You attract to you the predominant thoughts that you're holding in your awareness, whether those thoughts are conscious or unconscious." That means that in order to attract weight loss, you have to believe it on a conscious and subconscious level.

Here are a few examples. Your conscious mind may think "I hate the way my body looks and I really want to lose weight." However, your subconscious mind may think "I don't deserve to be happy. I am worthless. I need to be overweight to prove this." The result is that you will not lose weight. This subconscious thought is not something you are aware of but may be the result of messages you received as a child and have been acting on ever since. This is why willpower is not enough.

While not everyone has such deeply rooted self-sabotaging thoughts, most of us have thoughts about food and exercise that are not helping us. Sometimes, it's as simple as changing your thoughts about the things you need to do to be healthy and lose weight: focusing on what you love about healthy food, instead of what you are missing by not eating that cookie; or learning how to be calm and breathe through a moment of stress or sadness so that you don't give in to emotional eating; or thinking about how much you love, love, love exercise and how amazing and energized it makes you feel instead of "Ugh, I have to work out today."

The work is aligning your subconscious thoughts with your goals and reprogramming your subconscious mind to act on messages that help you to lose weight, not gain it or keep it on.

There are a few ways to achieve this, and I have found that hypnosis is the most effective.

Hypnosis is not what you see in the movies or on television. It's not mind control or voodoo. Hypnosis is relaxation. That's it! Ideally, you will feel like you are in the state between being awake and being asleep. After their first sessions, most of my clients say, "I don't feel like I was hypnotized!" This is because there is a preconceived notion of what hypnosis is based on its portrayal in the entertainment industry and stage shows. Clients do, however, say, "I was so relaxed," "I felt like I took a very long, refreshing nap" (even after a mere twenty-minute session), or "I felt like I was drifting and your voice sounded like it was far away." All of these are typical responses to a hypnosis experience. I've worked with clients in person and remotely all over the country, and no one has ever said they didn't feel in control or that they were not aware of what was happening. And no one has ever revealed their deep dark secrets to me during a session.

Hypnosis is not scary, but it is life-changing. It is not a magic cure, but it is an important weight loss tool. You are what you think. You must think that you deserve to be healthy and happy. You must think that you are in control of cravings and that you love moving your body and that you love eating nutrient-dense foods. You must visualize your ideal self, in mind, body, and spirit. Your subconscious mind is *the* secret!

Hypnosis success depends on lots of factors, two of which are repetition and positivity. For example, I never use the word *smoking* or *cigarette* for someone who wants to quit smoking; if I did, that's what her subconscious mind would focus on. Instead, I describe how much better her life will be when she instead becomes an air breather (the replacement term for non-smoker). The same is true for weight loss. Your mind must focus on all of the benefits and wonderful, glorious tastes of healthy foods and how amazing you feel when you work out. You must visualize success and how you want to look and feel. You have to believe it on every level of your being.

A few ways you can experience this repetition and positivity in your everyday life are through mantras and affirmations and changing your self-talk. One very simple example is using "I will" or "I am" instead of "I want to" or "I will try to." For example, "I will work out tomorrow," not "I'll try to work out tomorrow." I never let my clients tell me they will try. They will! Instead of

"I'm going to try not snacking after dinner," you say, "I'm not going to eat after dinner," or, even better, "I'm going to drink soothing warm lemon water if I feel hungry after dinner." This last phrase allows you to focus on what you are getting, not what you are giving up. Instead of "I want to lose ten pounds," it's "I am going to rock losing ten pounds! It's easy and fun!" Instead of "I really love doughnuts," say "I love eating fruit for breakfast. It's so refreshing and gives me energy." Your mind believes what you tell it over and over. If you tell yourself that you are so miserable because you can't have that pizza, your mind will believe you and you will be miserable. If you tell yourself that you love eating vegetables with every meal because they are so delicious and make you feel good, your mind will believe you and you will love eating vegetables with every meal. Give your mind the messages it needs to succeed!

This is an exercise you can do on your own and it is worth taking the time to do it. Pay attention to your self-talk as it relates to your weight, diet, exercise, and your goals. Write down the thoughts and intentions you have. Then reframe them to be positive and replace "will tries" and "wants" with "wills"! When you have your list, take all of the reframed thoughts and make them mantras that you repeat to yourself over and over. Put them on sticky notes throughout your house. Record them on your phone and listen to them on the way to work.

Journaling is also a very useful tool for recognizing and changing your thoughts. Being aware of the counterproductive thoughts you have about your body and weight and changing them to thoughts that serve you is an exercise I encourage in my program. Free association journaling about your body and weight loss also allows you to notice some recurring thoughts you are having that you may not even have realized existed! You are thinking all of the time. About your body. About food and exercise. About your weight. About your health. You have to become aware of these thoughts, and then work toward changing them. This is how journaling can help.

The word *yet* is a powerful word in this process. Every time you have a negative thought about your current state, add the word *yet* at the end. I do not fit into my size "x" pants … yet. My body is not in good shape … yet. I have no energy … yet. *Yet* is a guide to the future and a promise to get there. *Yet* is hope and your commitment to yourself and this journey.

In addition to your reframed thoughts, add some motivational quotes and affirmations to your list. Here are some examples:

- I feel healthy
- I am energetic
- I love moving my body
- I love eating fruits and vegetables
- I love drinking water

- I eat only what I need
- I love to exercise every day
- I am full of life
- I'm so lucky that I get to eat nutritious foods (can put in specific foods you plan to eat that day)
- I can do this
- I am strong in mind and body
- I am in control of my body and my mind
- I deserve to be happy and healthy
- Every day I feel lighter and healthier
- It is easy to eat healthy foods
- I am grateful for my body
- I weigh (goal weight) pounds
- Losing weight is fun
- I think before I eat
- I love eating slowly and mindfully
- I am grateful I have a body that is able to exercise
- I love discovering delicious new foods that nourish my body
- I exercise because it makes me feel great
- I am slim and fit
- I always take care of my body
- I am healthy, focused, and determined
- I love myself

You may be thinking that this just seems too simplistic. However, sometimes it's the simple things that have the greatest impact! Your thoughts have to be aligned with your goals in order for you to succeed. This is a fact. Changing your thoughts and adding these mantras to your life is not time-consuming, but it will make a huge difference. I promise you! If you change your mind, you will change your life.

Chapter Eight

Be Grateful, Be Mindful

*"The vibration of gratitude attracts more positive things
into your life."*
– Cherie Roe Dirksen

*"Mindfulness is a way of befriending ourselves,
and our experience."*
– Jon Kabat-Zinn

Be Grateful

I am grateful to be writing this book. I am grateful that I get to come into your life to help you during this important, transformational time. I am grateful to do the work that I do. I am grateful for the computer I'm using at this moment to write this book. I'm grateful for the clothes I'm wearing. I'm grateful for the comfy couch I'm sitting on. I'm grateful for the green tea I'm sipping. I'm grateful that my kids are sleeping and my house is quiet!

Gratitude. Is. Powerful. When you are grateful, you are energetically in a good place to achieve your goals. Umm, what the what does this mean? Research consistently shows that gratitude = happiness. And I will tell you right now, it's difficult for sad people to be healthy. Depressed people don't lose weight. You have to be in a mentally and emotionally healthy place to be physically healthy. This is why a weight loss program that focuses on the mind and body is necessary for immediate *and* lasting change to occur. Gratitude helps you to notice all of the things in your life that are going well. It is a very powerful practice!

There are many different ways you can practice gratitude, and I've listed them below.

1. Keep a gratitude journal.

This can be a paper and pen version or even an ongoing list on your phone, tablet, or computer. At the end of each day, you make note of ten things that you are grateful for from your day.

2. Set a gratitude timer.

You can set a timer on your phone or in your home to go off a few times each day. Every time it goes off, it's a reminder to think of something you are grateful for at that moment.

3. Make a gratitude jar (my favorite).

This is a particularly useful one if you have kids because they can participate, too! Designate a jar or container in your home to be your gratitude jar. You can even have the kids decorate it! Each day, write down one or two things you are grateful for on a slip of paper, and place it into the jar. The psychological effect of seeing it fill up, and eventually seeing a full jar of all the things you are grateful for, is very impactful!

4. Keep a gratitude rock or small charm or item in your pocket.

Each time you remember it's there or touch it throughout your day, think of something you are grateful for.

5. Write a gratitude letter.

This is about going beyond yourself, and doing something nice for someone else, which will bring happiness back to you! Write a letter or email to someone in your life who you are grateful for and tell them why.

6. Take a gratitude walk.

If you are an outdoor girl like me, you will love this one. Leave your phone at home and take a walk, even if it's only for five to ten minutes, and spend that time only reflecting on what you are grateful for in your life.

All of these ideas force you to notice wonderful people, things, and acts in your life that you otherwise wouldn't because you are worrying about something, or thinking about your to-do list, or on your phone. Having a gratitude practice will make you a happier person. And happy people want to be healthy, and they are able to take the steps necessary to be healthy and lose weight. No matter what your life circumstances are, you have things to be grateful for. It can be as simple as "I'm grateful for the opportunity to wake up this morning" to "I'm grateful I have my eyesight and can read this book" to "I'm grateful for the vacation I get to take with my kids this summer" or "I'm grateful for these berries I'm going to feed to my kids and myself" (wink wink).

Speaking of the berries, practicing gratitude also helps you to be thankful for the nourishment your body is receiving. As I discussed in chapter 1, having this positive relationship with food is extremely important. Food is not the enemy. Eating food that nourishes and energizes you and being grateful for the nutrition it is providing your body is a wonderful habit to put in place. Be grateful for its taste and all the flavors you are experiencing. You will also learn to appreciate that you are able to afford this food, and feed it to your children. This is a great lesson to teach your kids as well, at every meal. Say thank you for the food you are eating. Explain how and why it is nourishing their body and mind. I always spend time at dinner explaining why I'm feeding them the food that I am—this has protein and makes you strong, this has lots of vitamins to help your brain work so you can learn at school, etc. Encourage them to experience gratitude for the food they are consuming. You don't have to be religious or thank anyone specific if that is not your thing. Just put into place an experience of gratitude at every meal. It takes practice, but if you do it every day, for just a few minutes, you will notice that your food choices will slowly change. You will naturally make choices that you know will nourish your body and mind because you are practicing gratitude for them, and it's hard to feel grateful for something that you know will make you sick. Making the effort to change your thinking and practice gratitude will change your weight, your health, and your life.

Another benefit of practicing gratitude is stress relief. When you are stressed, it affects your body in many ways. Many of my clients who have come to me to lose weight admit having a habit of stress-eating, and usually it's not because they are hungry, and usually it's not fruits and veggies that they are binging on. In these cases, stress is directly leading to weight gain.

Even if you are not a stress-eater, stress has a systemic, negative effect on all of your being. It affects your sleep quality, your experience of joy and happiness, your ability to make healthy choices, and even your gut health, which you now know leads to weight gain (or difficulty losing weight), inflammation, and chronic disease.

So how can you use gratitude to manage stress? Imagine how differently you would feel if every time you felt stressed about all of the laundry you had to do, you instead think "I'm grateful that my kids have clothing to wear," or every time your sink was full of dishes, you think "I'm grateful to have dirty plates, because that means that my kids ate today." Simple but powerful.

Just. Be. Grateful. Don't just say you are grateful. Be grateful. Feel it, experience it, practice it, mean it.

Be Mindful

Gratitude and mindfulness go hand in hand, and here is why. To be grateful, you have to be mindful. Mindfulness refers to being in the present moment and experiencing it, without judgment. When you do that, you will discover what you are grateful for in that moment. You can't be grateful and distracted at the same time. You must be aware, mindful, in the present moment. Mindfulness also contributes to a less stressful, happier life experience. When you are in the moment, you will experience a calm and sense of peace that most moms find difficult to find in everyday life. For example, I come home from work and usually think about how I have to take my dog out, get everyone from school and the bus stop, clean up, start preparing dinner, etc, etc, etc. You know the drill. But when I practice mindfulness, I'm in the moment with my kids, enjoying that moment. Not thinking or worrying about *anything* else. Even if there is chaos around me, I can go be with my kids and have a conversation with them or give them a hug or just smile at them and be in that moment.

Mindfulness is very important when in the throes of weight loss. Veronica was a client in my weight loss program who had one very rough night where everything seemed to be going wrong—she overcooked her dinner and had nothing else to eat. She had a rough day and was in a very negative mindset. However, she remembered to take a step back. She stopped, was present in the moment, thought of what she had to be grateful for, and then moved forward with her evening, feeling more centered and less stressed. Although she was still hungry and disappointed in her dinner fail, she was able to handle it from a better state of mind and could appreciate what she could learn from the situation.

I also teach my clients to be mindful during workouts. When we do group workouts online, I always remind them to think about the muscles they are strengthening in that exact moment. I remind them to pay attention to their heart working so hard and how their body is pumping endorphins through their body. It's a very meaningful experience to be with your body in that moment, experiencing gratitude for what it's doing for you to help you lose weight. This is a much better practice than thinking about how hard it is, or wanting it to be over because it hurts too much. Focusing on how you are getting stronger and burning calories at that exact moment actually makes the time go faster!

That's how mindfulness works. Be in the present moment. Be aware of it. Love it. Appreciate it.

Teach your kids to be mindful. Teach them to take deep breaths. Teach them to stop and smell the roses. This comes more naturally to children anyway, but at some point, it starts to fade away; this is where you can be the good example. Being mindful and grateful will make you happier and calmer, and even healthier, but it is a practice that will also provide a good example for your kids. Having these skills will allow them to navigate life's challenges a lot more successfully. It's a win-win (win-win-win, depending on how many kids you have).

Chapter Nine
Don't Worry, Be Happy

*"Happiness cannot be traveled to, owned, earned, worn,
or consumed. Happiness is the spiritual experience of
living every minute with love, grace, and gratitude."*
– Denis Waitley

I realize that *happiness* is a very subjective term. What does it really mean to be happy? I think this is different for everyone, but in general, it means being mindful and grateful, experiencing moments of joy and holding on to them, tapping into your strengths to get through difficulties, having a purpose to work toward that brings you a sense of meaning, having a social support system, and feeling excited to get out of bed in the morning to experience all that the universe has to offer you. When you experience happiness, you want to eat nutritious foods and exercise, because you love and appreciate your body and you want to take care of it.

So, how do you achieve happiness? First, you have to be ready to accept happiness. You have to believe that you deserve it. You must really believe it. You deserve to be happy. Just like your children deserve to be happy, so do you. You cannot achieve happiness unless you know that you deserve it. Say it over and over: "I deserve to be happy." Say it until you believe it. All day, every day.

Joyful Moments

Life is full of joy, happiness, and love. You just have to be mindful enough to notice it. When you practice mindfulness, and are fully in the moment, you can appreciate the joy of that moment. No past to dwell on, no future to worry about. Just be in a moment. When you are at the park with your kids, how joyful it is to be outside, getting fresh air and being able to take your kids somewhere safe where they can play. Look up, close your eyes, breathe in the joy of life. When you are cooking dinner and your kids are screaming, you can even find joy in that moment. How lucky you are that your kids have a voice to express themselves and that you have food to cook for them. Stop, be in the moment, smile. There is always something to feel joyful about.

Another way to experience joy is to write down all of the activities, thoughts, and memories that bring you joy and happiness. Do them or think of them often. Set reminders or carry them with you until it becomes habit. Make sticky notes with positive words on them to post around your home (joy, love, gratitude, serenity, hope, inspiration, pride, interest, fun, peace). Read your gratitude lists. Look at pictures or watch videos of happy memories. Allow yourself to feel what you felt in these moments. Don't let it go. Allow it to become part of you. Tap into it often.

Strengths

You are a unique, amazing person who has strengths that you probably don't even realize. Your weight-loss journey is a powerful process that will help you recognize how strong you really are! I want you to know what your strengths are so that you can use them when you need to.

So, what are your strengths? Here are some questions you can ask yourself:

- What am I naturally good at?
- What kinds of tasks am I naturally drawn toward?
- What would my ideal job be?
- What do I enjoy doing most?
- What play scenarios did I repeat over and over as a child?
- Now think about a difficult time you have gone through.
- What inside of yourself did you tap into to get through it?

- What did you draw from to overcome it?

Answering these questions will allow you to understand what your strengths are. Write them down. Now, when you are going through something challenging, or you wake up in the morning and aren't feeling it today, look at this list. How can you use these strengths to overcome and not just push through, but thrive? You are amazing and unique. You are strong. You are capable of doing anything you put your mind to.

You can also use this list to thrive at this weight-loss process! For example, if you are an organized person who enjoys lists and planning, this will work in your favor when it's time to plan meals, schedule workouts, and write grocery lists! If you are a creative person, you can use that creativity to come up with fun recipes and ways to involve your kids in cooking with you. If sociability is one of your strengths, you can use this to organize a weight-loss group in your area, or find a friend in a workout class to be your workout buddy.

Whatever your strengths are, use them. Nurture them. Cultivate them. Take full advantage of them every day.

Purpose and Meaning

Happy people have purpose and meaning, and not just one. It's a misconception that you have to have this one big meaning in your life. Your purpose changes, and you can find many different ways to find meaning throughout your life. Some of your current purposes may be raising your kids, doing a good job at work, making money to support your family, or volunteering with animals or the environment. These things bring you meaning. Taking care of yourself is also one of your purposes.

You may also have a purpose that you haven't discovered yet. If you feel like something is missing and you can't quite put your finger on it, it may be that you have a purpose waiting for you! Think about what causes and issues make you feel inspired or excited. Look at your list of strengths and figure out how you can utilize them for your happiness and for the greater good. What are you good at, what are you passionate about, and how can you combine these two in ways that makes you excited to get out of bed in the morning?

For me, it was my career. I absolutely love helping people be their best selves. My job is one of my passions and purposes, and so is raising my children. Raising my children is literally what gets me out of bed every day, but my job is what makes me jump out of bed, happy and excited to start the day. I don't feel guilty saying this, because I love my kids more than anything, but parenting is not easy. I'm able to find the moments of joy in everyday life, and they get to experience a mom who is joyful because she found a purpose that brings her meaning. My hope is that they will always be inspired to do the same.

Your purpose does not have to be grandiose. It can be creating art that you enjoy reading or looking at. It can be volunteering a few hours a month for a cause that is meaningful to you. It can be organizing social events among your neighbors and your group of friends to bring people together. Whatever it is, take the time to discover it, practice it, and nurture it. We all deserve to be happy and to enjoy getting out of bed in the morning. Find a purpose that brings you a sense of meaning.

Find Your People

Happy people have other people. Even if you are an introvert or "loner," find one person to be your person.

I have found over and over again that people who succeed in losing weight over the long term have found their people. They have people to support them, inspire them, motivate them, and hold them accountable. They have people with whom they can be very honest about their life struggles and how they are feeling. Usually this is a mix of professionals (health coaches, personal trainers, group exercise instructors, etc.), and friends and family. Even an online forum or support group can be effective, but you must have people.

And not just people, but people who really love and support you. Not people who create drama, and make you feel bad about yourself. Not people who are there for you when it's convenient for them or because of what they get out of the relationship. Find the relationships that lift you up, inspire you, and motivate you to be your best self and nurture them. Give them your time and attention.

Start to pay attention to how you feel when you are with the people in your life. Notice if you feel agitated, defensive, on edge, nervous, sad, or if you feel excited, peaceful, calm, and like your true self. Surround yourself with people who make you feel good, who love you for exactly who you are, and who will support you through this journey, because they know you would do the same for them. These are the people worth taking this life journey with. As a mom, your time is precious. You have so many commitments, and you are now making one to yourself. Don't waste your very precious time with people who don't lift you up. You are amazing and beautiful, and everyone you choose to surround yourself with should remind you of this.

I run my weight loss program in a group format for several reasons. The main one is that the support of other powerful women and moms on the same journey is extraordinarily transformative. Being able to share your struggles and help other people through theirs allows you to know that you are not alone. Each group I run is unique and special because of the people in them, who often form strong bonds that go beyond the twelve-week program.

Sarah was a client who told me she felt it was the social support of the group that really got her through. She had tried to do it alone or with one professional guide, but it didn't stick. She thrived on having the energy of others supporting her, holding her accountable, cheering her on, and encouraging her on bad days. Sarah attributed her final success to having her people.

Find. Your. People.

Chapter Ten

Meditation

*"The goal of meditation isn't to control your thoughts, it's
to stop letting them control you."*
– Unknown

I already know what you are thinking, and not because I'm
psychic, but because it's the number one response I get from
clients when I suggest meditation. It's always some version
of "I can't do that because I can't quiet my mind. I can't stop
thinking. I have too many thoughts. I'm bad at meditation."
Having thoughts is normal! We can't just turn off our thoughts.
Imagine how much simpler life would be if we could just decide
to shut down our brain whenever we wanted a much-needed
break from our worries and to-do lists. Meditation is not about
turning off your thoughts. It's about acknowledging them, and
letting them go. This is what happens when you first start meditating, and you grow from there.

Meditation is a spiritual practice that affects all levels of your being. I like to think of meditation like strength-training for the mind and spirit. You can't expect to go to the gym for the first time and leave forty pounds lighter and with a six-pack. Imagine if that was the expectation everyone had. Of course everyone would give up right away! Having a meaningful meditation practice takes practice. You can start with just one or two minutes. Most of that time will be spent acknowledging and letting go of your thoughts. But just like anything else, the more you practice, the easier it becomes, and the more benefits you will experience.

So what is the point of meditation? It's different for everyone, but since you are reading this book, I'm assuming that you would like to know how to use meditation to lose weight. So here goes.

One of the most important benefits of regular meditation is stress reduction. Raise your hand if you currently are or have ever been guilty of stress eating? Right! It's very common. In fact, it's what triggers many of my clients to give in to a craving for unhealthy foods. Besides unhealthy eating, stress has very detrimental effects on all levels of your being. It has been linked to heart disease, high blood pressure, insomnia, digestive issues, headaches, fertility problems, sexual dysfunction, depression, and anxiety. Doesn't having a practice in place—one that involves just sitting for a few minutes a day and being still (a mom's dream come true)—that will also help you to live a longer and healthier life sound awesome?

There are many kinds of meditation that you can practice. There are a few that are more useful for weight loss. One is guided meditation. Guided meditation is when you are coached by someone else's words to imagine something. Your imagination is very powerful. (It is also what hypnosis taps into.) Guided meditation for weight loss may involve you focusing on your goal weight, how you want to look and feel, or imagining yourself going through a typical day with the diet and exercise you need to do. This is a good way to start a meditation practice, because it is "easier" since your mind has something to focus on. There are many apps, websites, and videos online that offer guided meditation recordings that you can use for weight loss. In my weight loss program, I offer personalized meditations and we do group meditations weekly. Encouraging my clients to meditate regularly helps them to stay centered and focused on their goals.

You can also use mantra meditation, which is a type of meditation in which you repeat a mantra over and over. You can choose one of your weight loss mantras that is applicable to you at that moment or that you feel connected to. Why are mantras and mantra meditation effective? According to Giovanni Dienstmann,

"A mantra replaces 10,000 different thoughts by one thought—a thought that gives peace and awareness. It allows you to collect your scattered attention, which is spread thin all over the place, and unify it, thus empowering it."

By repeating a mantra, you are not only aligning energetically with that phrase, but you are using all of your mind power to focus on one thing, which is very powerful—especially when this one thing is exactly what you need to lose weight. Mantra meditation also naturally helps your mind stay on track and not wander to other things.

Mindfulness meditation is what most people think of when they say, "Meditation is hard." This is the type of meditation that involves sitting with just your thoughts, being fully aware in the present moment and allowing yourself to just be. I use the Just Be exercise in workshops and with clients, and you can try it now! Set a timer, close your eyes, and just be, for one minute. Then notice, where did your thoughts go, how did you feel, and why? Practice this often!

Mindfulness meditation is important for weight loss because it helps you to practice being fully aware and present in each moment. This is useful for stress management and managing emotions that may lead to emotional eating. It's also helpful when you have cravings. If you can't stop thinking about eating a cupcake, come back to the present moment, breathe through it, just be. Give that obsessive thought permission to leave. Replace it with gratitude. Then move on. The more you practice mindfulness meditation, the more you train your brain how to be mindful. Being mindful in your everyday life makes you happier, more joyful, and better equipped to get through cravings and stressful moments.

So, now you may be thinking, "How do I start a meditation practice?" First, like exercise and meal-planning, choose a time each day. Some people like to start the day with meditation; some like to end it by meditating. You decide and set aside that time. For purposes of staying awake, I do recommend sitting up, in a comfortable position. However, you can practice while lying down if you prefer. Then you either listen to a recording of a guided meditation on your phone or computer, or practice mantra or mindfulness meditation as described above. The key is committing to it, and making it a priority. Make it part of your weight loss plan and treat it with equal importance to diet and exercise, because it is.

Beth was a client of mine who was very good at stress eating. When she experienced stress, she automatically went for junk food. We worked to implement a mindfulness and meditation practice to reduce stress. When paired with hypnosis, this was very effective in helping her make different choices and experience less stress!

Learning to calm your mind instead of focusing on all of the thoughts that aren't serving you is very powerful. Doing so leads to an ongoing, calmer state of being where you feel more centered and better able to handle stressors that arise, instead of automatically reacting according to old habits and patterns, such as stress eating.

Meditation is something that schools and programs are using more and more for children. This is one of those weight loss-tools that you can absolutely incorporate into parenting. A 2016 Forbes article listed the benefits that children who practiced meditation experienced, and they included increased focus and attention, better attendance and higher grades in school, a decrease in anxiety and depression, being more self-aware and practicing self-regulation, and more responsible decision-making and prosocial behavior. While I recommend having a meditation practice just for you, I also recommend having one that you do with your children. Practice every night before bed right after you read them a story or talk about their day. Do it together for five minutes. This is just as beneficial to their overall health and development as eating vegetables for dinner. And all it involves is sitting in silence for a few minutes!

So, to recap, meditation is a spiritual practice that involves sitting still for a few minutes each day, can help you to lose weight, can prevent disease, and can help your kids live happier and healthier lives. What are you waiting for?

Chapter Eleven

Manifest Your Awesome Self

*"The Law of Attraction is always working, whether you
believe it or understand it or not."*
– Bob Proctor, *The Secret*

The law of attraction. It's powerful, perhaps the most powerful force in the universe. And you can use it to lose weight and be healthy. The law of attraction (LOA) already dictates your life experiences through your thoughts. I want to teach you how to use it to dictate your health and weight loss.

The law of attraction is quite simple to understand and apply: like attracts like. So, if you are thinking negative thoughts most of the time, what are you going to attract? Negativity. On the flip side, if you can be mindful and train your mind to think positive thoughts that focus on what you want, you will attract positivity and your dreams will come true! Sounds too good to be true, I know. But it's simply quantum physics. Your thoughts are like magnets. What you think, you attract, good or bad. You are always, always thinking. Most of the time, you are not even aware that you are thinking or what you are thinking of. This is why mindfulness is key. Learning to be mindful of your thoughts is the first step in changing them.

Now that you understand the LOA and how it works, you can start doing it! Here are some powerful ways to tap into it.

1. Make a vision board, or two, or three.

This is the very first task I give new clients. They come to our first meeting with a completed vision board. A vision board is a board that you create, either with poster board and images from the internet, magazines, etc. or there are many websites now that allow you to make vision boards online to print or look at on your computer. I'm a big proponent of having it somewhere physically in your home rather than just on your computer. However, if you spend a lot of time on your computer for work, then having it there is also useful.

Your vision board is your vision of exactly what you want to achieve in life. So if your goal is to lose weight, your vision board will contain images of slim and toned bodies, sneakers as a reminder to exercise, the bathing suit or outfit you want to wear, the foods you want to eat, the words, phrases, and quotes that inspire and motivate you, the vacation you want to take. You can also post the number of pounds you want to lose or your goal weight. When it's finished you place it somewhere in your home where you will see it all of the time. For weight loss, the kitchen is a good choice. You can also choose to make more than one for other rooms in your home, for your car, your office, etc. When you look at these images all day, this is what your mind will focus on, and this is what you will attract to you. When you visualize it, so it will be.

Additionally, this is something you can get your kids involved in! Ask them to help you with yours or to make their own!

Christina was a client who was very into vision boards. She made one on poster board for her kitchen, and one on her phone that she could look at all day. She would always say that focusing on these images helped her to stay attuned to her goals, especially during moments when she had cravings. She felt very strongly that these images allowed her to stay on track and gave her a sense of accomplishment.

This is an awesome example of how vision boards can work for you on this journey. Focusing on images that represent health and weight loss to you will naturally cause you to make decisions that will get you those outcomes

2. Be grateful every day for your thin, healthy body.

Practice gratitude, but not just for what you have now. The LOA works when you are living the life you want in your mind already. So in your mind, be your goal weight and size and be grateful for it. Several times a day, say to yourself, "Thank you for this thin, healthy body." In addition, thank your food. Every single time you put a nutritious food or drink in your body, say to yourself, "Thank you for keeping me thin and healthy." I realize that can sound crazy. For real, I get it. But this is how it works! I'm not making it up; I'm just relaying it to you. Be grateful for being thin and healthy, and so it will be!

3. Think thin.

Identify any "fat thoughts,"—any negative thoughts you have about your body—and replace them with "My body is perfect" and "I love my body." You have to love your body to lose weight. When you love your body, you are motivated to take care of it. Your body works so hard for you. Love it, appreciate it, think of your body in a positive way. Practice self-love and acceptance through mantras and affirmations until you believe it. When you believe it, so it will be.

4. Live your day as your ideal self.

How will your life be different when you lose this weight? Walk around as if you are your ideal weight or size. How would you approach life differently? How would your day be different? How would you present yourself? Will you walk taller, smile more, have more energy? How would you feel? Live this life. Attract it to you with every thought and action. When you live it, so it will be.

5. Visualize before sleep.

Every night before you go to sleep, imagine yourself standing in a full-length mirror and your image being exactly what you want it to be: size, weight, clothing, skin, with as much detail as possible. Your reflection is smiling, she is glowing, she is thin, she is healthy, she is you. Fall asleep with this image in your mind. When you see it and dream it, so it will be.

I'll say again, I realize that some of these may make seem too simplistic or a little out there, but this is just how the LOA works. The reason not everyone is using it is because they don't believe it works, and they think these things sound outlandish and hippy-ish and new age–ish. But what if it does work? What if, just what if, you chose to commit yourself to these small changes and you lost all of the weight you wanted to? Wouldn't it be worth trying? What do you have to lose?

The answer: all of the weight you have been holding on to. What do you have to gain? The answer: lifelong health and wellness, energy to be with your kids, presence of mind to enjoy being a mom, a role model your kids can look up to and learn from, and a healthier, happier you!

Chapter Twelve
Let's Do This

Are you ready to do this? By now, you know that weight loss and ongoing wellness is a holistic process, and that with time, commitment, planning, and the right mindset, you can achieve it!

Here are the next steps to creating your weight loss plan:

1. Start drinking a green smoothie every day and focus on creating a diet and meal plan that contains mostly whole foods.

2. Make a weekly plan—meals, shopping list, and days you will work out.

3. Create good sleep habits.

4. Write down some mantras, either from chapter 7 or ones that you create. Write them on sticky notes, record them on your phone, and say them to yourself all day long.

5. Choose a gratitude practice to implement with you and your kids!

6. Start being mindful, living in the moment, and becoming aware of your thoughts.

7. Notice and savor joyful moments! Acknowledge your strengths and find something that gives you a sense of meaning and purpose.

8. Journal about your feelings on your body and what thoughts have prevented you from losing weight so far. Become aware of your self-talk and identify self-sabotaging thoughts like "I will never lose weight," or "I know I won't be able to do it," or "I don't have time to exercise." Reframe them to be positive, such as "I love losing weight," "I am strong and can do anything I put my mind to," and "I love finding time to exercise."

9. Find supportive people and someone to hold you accountable.

10. Practice meditation.

11. Create a vision board to manifest health and weight loss.

This is the weight loss program I guide my clients through, and this is what works!

Even after you do all of this, it's important to understand that wellness is an ongoing process. That's why it's critical to your success to have support and accountability when starting a weight-loss program. Once you have these habits established over a period of weeks, it's easier for you to maintain them and carry them forward successfully on your own. This is also why dieting and exercise alone don't always work. You have to know how to be in the right mindset of health. Learn how to manage stress and challenging emotions. Learn how to use the LOA for health and other life goals. Teach your family these skills as well and hold each other accountable.

My wish for you is for you to understand that weight loss is not just a diet and exercise plan, but a holistic process that can be learned and enjoyed! Just like everything else in life, it is a learning experience. You can use it to learn more about yourself and how strong you really are if you choose to do so. Viewing it in this way makes it a challenge to overcome—an opportunity to realize how strong you really are! Seeing the bigger picture and viewing challenges in this way leaves opportunities for growth and transformation beyond your wildest dreams!

I also encourage you to talk to your kids about this journey. Let them see you work hard toward an important goal. Let them know you are doing it for them and for yourself. Let them help you through difficult moments and celebrate your successes, just like you do for them! Allow them to be part of the process. Teach them how to be healthy and to use their mind to achieve their goals. This new lifestyle is for everyone. This new mindset will benefit your entire family.

You will have bad days, you will feel like quitting, you will want to go on a cake binge. But guess what, you will also overcome, you will realize how strong you really are, you will be healthy and lose weight, you will be an inspiration for your kids, family, and friends. You will do this!

Recommended Reading

The 21-Day Belly Fix: The Doctor-Designed Diet Plan for a Clean Gut and a Slimmer Waist by Dr. Tasneem Bhatia

Clean Gut by Alejandro Junger

Your Mind: The Owner's Manual by LindaJoy Rose

Raw Fusion: Better Living Through Living Foods by LindaJoy Rose

Acknowledgments

This book would never have been written without the education I received at the Natural Wellness Academy. Finding the NWA changed my life, and has allowed me to do a job I love and live a life of my dreams. To my mentor, LindaJoy Rose, for her guidance and patience, her knowledge and passion, thank you.

To the Morgan James Publishing team: Special thanks to David Hancock, CEO & Founder for believing in me and my message. To my Author Relations Manager, Margo Toulouse, thanks for making the process seamless and easy. Many more thanks to everyone else, but especially Jim Howard, Bethany Marshall, and Nickcole Watkins.

To L, for inspiring me to want to eat the berries.

To my parents and brother, who have always been there for me—to support me, clean my house, watch my kids and dogs, and love me even when I'm crazy.

To my entire family for being the people I love coming home to.

To my village, for helping me to get through this crazy ride called parenting. For carpooling my kids, for letting me cry, for keeping me company, for making me laugh so hard I cry, for dancing, for bringing me wine, for loving me. I could not do it without you.

To my clients, who inspire me and motivate me to be better.

To D, my rock-and-roll partner on this journey, thank you for asking me to be with you twenty-seven years ago and not giving up on me since. Life is better with you in it. I love you.

To my kids, for giving me the best job in the world. For showing me how strong I am, teaching me patience, and inspiring me to take care of myself so that I can take care of you. For loving me on my bad days and good ones, and for all the hugs, kisses, and cuddles that make life so joyful. I love you to the moon and back.

About the Author

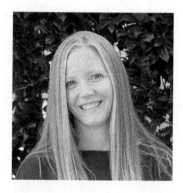

Jamie Hernandez earned a bachelor degree from Penn State University in human development and family studies and two master's degrees from New York University in psychology and counseling. She has always had a passion for helping people to become the best versions of themselves. In her career, she has worked with children with developmental delays and provided college counseling for high school students and drug and alcohol counseling for people in recovery.

Her passion for health and wellness started in 2008 with the birth of her first child. When she discovered the field of holistic health coaching, she was excited to merge her passions for helping others and for wellness into a career. Jamie received certifications as a holistic health and life coach and a hypnotherapist from the Natural Wellness Academy, where she continues to create new courses and mentor students to follow their dreams of helping others.

Jamie is the mother of four beautiful children and specializes in helping other busy moms to achieve holistic health and wellness. Jamie knows that moms are the core of their families, and that when she teaches moms to be healthy, the entire family will benefit.

Jamie also has a passion for animal rescue and welfare. She is currently raising two rescue pups and regularly donates to animal rescue causes.

Email: jamiehealthcoach@gmail.com

Website: www.wholefoodspirit.com

Facebook Page: Jamie Hernandez, Holistic Health Coach & Hypnotherapist

Pinterest: Whole Food & Spirit

Thank You

As my thanks to you, my fellow awesome mom, I want to inspire and motivate you to take care of yourself. Therefore, I invite you to join me on my weight loss support group on Facebook. This is where I post my weight loss tips, answer questions, and do live webinars to educate and inspire you to take action and keep going!

Join me on Facebook at "Eat the Berries: Weight Loss for Busy Moms" to stay connected with me, and so I can connect with you!

https://www.facebook.com/groups/weightlossforrealbusy-moms/

CPSIA information can be obtained
at www.ICGtesting.com
Printed in the USA
LVHW031740030619
619985LV00003B/579/P